RVT & Veterinary Assistant Job Aid

RVT & Veterinary Assistant Job Aid

TaLethia, RVT, CBOM

Library of Congress Control Number: 2021915566
ISBN: Hardcover   978-1-6641-8747-4
                Softcover   978-1-6641-8746-7
                eBook   978-1-6641-8745-0

Print information available on the last page.

Rev. date: 07/29/2021

To order additional copies of this book, contact:
Xlibris
844-714-8691
www.Xlibris.com
Orders@Xlibris.com
828427

CONTENTS

Veterinary Technician Oath

I solemnly dedicate myself to aiding animals and society by providing excellent care and services for animals, by alleviating animal suffering, and promoting public health.

I accept my obligations to practice my profession conscientiously and with sensitivity, adhering to the profession's Code of Ethics, and furthering my knowledge and competence through a commitment to lifelong learning.

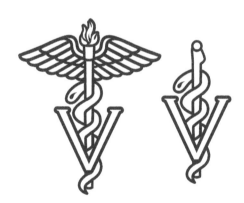

Normal Critical Values

Parameter	Canine	Feline	
Temperature (F)	99.5–102.5	100–102.5	
Heart rate (BPM)	70–180	145–200	
Respiratory rate (BPM)	20–40	20–40	
Capillary refill time (CRT) seconds	< 1.5	< 1.5	
Mucous membrane color	Pink	Pink	
Blood pressure (mmHg)—systolic	100–150	100–150	
Blood pressure (mmHg)—diastolic	60–110	60–110	
Mean arterial blood pressure (MAP)	80–120	80–120	
$ETCO_2$	> 40 mmHg Hyperventilating	< 30 mmHg Hyperventilating	
Packed cell volume (PCV) %	35–54	27–46	
Total plasma protein (TP) g/dl	5.7–7.3	6.3–8.3	
Blood urea nitrogen (BUN) mg/dl	8.0–25	15–35	
Urine output ml/kg/hr	1.0–2.0	1.0–2.0	
Creatinine mg/dl	0.5–1.3	1.0–2.2	
iCa (ionized calcium) mmol/l	1.12–1.40	1.20–1.32	
K (potassium) mmol/l	3.7–5.8	4.0–4.5	
Cl (chloride) mmol/l	105–115	117–123	
Na (sodium) mmol/l	140–159	147–156	
Glucose mg/dl	60–110	64–118	
PLT (platelets) × 100,000/ul	2.0–9.0	1.5–5.0	
ALB (albumin)	2.5–4.3	2.2–4.4	

1

Common Sedation, Anesthetic, and Emergency Drug Doses

Before using any of the following drugs, please refer to the prescribing DVM and Plumb's Veterinary Drug Handbook for treatment suggestions, contraindications, and/or potential adverse effects. Dose ranges are listed because a variety of doses have been published. Please note that the lowest and safest effective dose should be utilized. It is the practitioner's responsibility to know the current regulations regarding off-label use and to have appropriate consent and/or release forms signed prior to administration of any medication.

I have made every effort to ensure the accuracy of the information with regard to drug dosages and routes. However, appropriate information sources should be consulted, especially when new or unfamiliar drugs are first being utilized. It is the responsibility of every veterinarian and veterinary professional to evaluate the appropriateness of a particular opinion in the context of actual clinical situations and with due consideration to new developments and the patient whom the medication is being prescribed for.

Drug	Concentration	Dose	Route	Comments
Activated charcoal		3–5 ml/kg	PO	
Acepromazine	(Dilute) 1 mg/ml	0.02–0.05 mg/kg	IV	
Antisedan	5 mg/ml	0.15 ml/lb	IM	
Apomorphine	1 mg/ml	0.02–0.04 mg/kg	IV	
Apomorphine	1 mg/ml	0.25 mg	Conjunctiva	
Atropine	0.54 mg/ml	0.05 mg/kg	IV	
Blood	Units	10 ml/lb or 20 ml/kg	IV	
Buprenorphine (Buprenex)	0.3 mg/ml	0.005–0.01 mg/kg	IV	

Butorphanol (Torb)	10 mg/ml	0.2–0.5 mg/kg	IV	
Calcium gluconate	10% = 100 mg/ml	0.5–1.5 ml/kg	IV (slow)	Monitor w/ EKG during Tx
Dexamethasone SP	4 mg/ml	2.2–4.4 mg/kg	IV	
Dexdomitor— microdose	500 ug/ml	1–3 u/kg	IV	
Dexdomitor— regular dose	500 ug/ml	0.02 mg/kg	IV	
Diphenhydramine (Benadryl)	50 mg/ml	1–2 mg/kg	IV/SQ	
Epinephrine	1 mg/ml	1 ml/20 lb	IV	
Etomidate	2 mg/ml	1.5 mg/kg	IV	
Flumazenil	0.1 mg/ml	0.01 mg/kg	IV	
Glycopyrrolate	0.2 mg/ml	0.005–0.01 mg/kg	IV	
Hetastarch	6% = 60 mg/ml	20 ml/kg/24 hrs	IV infusion	DVM will Rx dose
Hydromorphone	2 mg/ml	0.1 mg/kg	IV/IM	
Ketamine/Valium	100 mg/ml & 5 mg/ml	1 ml / 20 lb	IV	Dilute 1:1
Lidocaine	2% = 20 mg/ml	2.2 mg/kg (bolus)	IV	Canine dose
Mannitol	200 mg/ml	1–2 g/kg	IV	Use filter to infuse
Midazolam	5 mg/ml	0.2 mg/kg	IV	
Morphine	2 mg/kg	0.1 mg/kg	IV	
Naloxone	0.4 mg/ml	0.03 mg/kg	IV	
Oxymorphone	1.5 mg/ml	0.2–0.2 mg/kg	IV	
Oxytocin	20 u/ml	Canine = max 20 u	IM	
Oxytocin	20 u/ml	Feline = max 1–3 u	IM	
Propofol (PropoFlo)	10 mg/ml	4–6 mg/kg	IV	
Sodium bicarbonate	1 mEq/ml = 84 mg/ml	1 mEq/kg	IV	
Whole blood	Single or double units	10 ml/lb	IV infusion	DVM will Rx dose
Xylazine	100 mg/ml	0.4 mg/kg	IM	DVM will Rx dose

3

Yohimbine	2 mg/ml	0.11 mg/kg	IV	DVM will Rx dose
External defibrillation	**Patient < 7 kg**	2 J/kg		
External defibrillation	Patient 8–40 kg	5 J/kg		
External defibrillation	**Patient > 40 kg**	5–10 J/kg		

Percent (%) Solution Calculation

% desired volume × volume desired
divided by
% stock solution on hand

Calculation = volume of stock solution
needed in ml to be added to base fluid

Note: You will need to subtract the difference of the stock solution
volume from the base solution to ensure proper dilution factor.

Example

2.5% needed to be created of dextrose in 1L bag for
an IV constant rate infusion (CRI) for a patient
In this example, dextrose is a 50% stock solution.

Calculation: 2.5% × 1,000 ml / 50% = 50 ml of the
stock dextrose solution to add to 1L of fluids

Note: You will need to **remove** 50 ml of the fluids from the
1L bag of IV fluids **before** adding the 50 ml of dextrose to
ensure the proper prescribed dilution factor strength.

TIP: Confirm with the DVM how often you will need to monitor
the patient's blood glucose (BG) and if the dextrose percentage
concentration will need to be adjusted pending the results.

*Please be aware there are many ways to calculate
dextrose percentages. This is just my favorite way.*

Doses of chemotherapeutic agents are often calculated on the basis of body surface area in square meters rather than by the kilogram weight.

The chart below provides the conversion from kilogram body weight to square meter surface area.

Body Surface Area Conversion Chart (Body Weight in Kilograms to Meters Squared)									
Weight to Body Surface Area Conversion Chart—Dogs									
kg	m^2	kg	m^2	kg	m^2	kg	m^2	kg	m^2
0.5	0.064	10.0	0.469	20.0	0.744	30.0	0.975	40.0	1.181
1.0	0.101	11.0	0.500	21.0	0.759	31.0	0.997	41.0	1.201
2.0	0.160	12.0	0.529	22.0	0.785	32.0	1.018	42.0	1.220
3.0	0.210	13.0	0.553	23.0	0.817	33.0	1.029	43.0	1.240
4.0	0.255	14.0	0.581	24.0	0.840	34.0	1.060	44.0	1.259
5.0	0.295	15.0	0.608	25.0	0.864	35.0	1.081	45.0	1.278
6.0	0.333	16.0	0.641	26.0	0.886	36.0	1.101	46.0	1.297
7.0	0.370	17.0	0.668	27.0	0.909	37.0	1.121	47.0	1.302
8.0	0.404	18.0	0.694	28.0	0.931	38.0	1.142	48.0	1.334
9.0	0.437	19.0	0.719	29.0	0.953	39.0	1.162	49.0	1.352
								50.0	1.371
Weight to Body Surface Area Conversion Chart—Cats									
kg	m^2	kg	m^2	kg	m^2	kg	m^2	kg	m^2
0.1	0.022	1.4	0.125	3.6	0.235	5.8	0.323	8.0	0.400
0.2	0.034	1.6	0.137	3.8	0.244	6.0	0.330	8.2	0.407

0.3	0.045	1.8	0.148	4.0	0.252	6.2	0.337	8.4	0.413
0.4	0.054	2.0	0.159	4.2	0.260	6.4	0.345	8.6	0.420
0.5	0.063	2.2	0.169	4.4	0.269	6.6	0.352	8.8	0.426
0.6	0.071	2.4	0.179	4.6	0.277	6.8	0.360	9.0	0.433
0.7	0.079	2.6	0.189	4.8	0.285	7.0	0.366	9.2	0.439
0.8	0.086	2.8	0.199	5.0	0.292	7.2	0.373	9.4	0.445
0.9	0.093	3.0	0.208	5.2	0.300	7.4	0.380	9.6	0.452
1.0	0.100	3.2	0.217	5.4	0.307	7.6	0.387	9.8	0.458
1.2	0.113	3.4	0.226	5.6	0.315	7.8	0.393	10.0	0.464

Scavenger Hunt for a Physical or Paper Patient Medical File

*Below is a list of true locations where I
have found charts or lab forms.
If you've lost a physical record, this list will help you find it.*

- *Primary filing system*
- *DVM desk*
- *Callback area*
- *To-be-filed area*
- *Next day's appointments*
- *Treatment room*
- *Procedure room*
- *Radiology*
- *Manager's office*
- *Hospitalized patient's chart holder*
- *Current day's appointment slot*
- *Exam room*
- *Secondary department*
- *Filed under wrong name (maiden name or hyphenated name)*
- *Previous year's filing system*
- *Bathroom*
- *Break room*
- *Deceased filing system*
- *Prescription-refill slot*
- *Top of cages*
- *Ready-to-discharge slot*
- *To-be-faxed or to-be-emailed slot*
- *Reception area / lobby*
- *Collections/accounts manager*
- *Outside*
- *In car or home of DVM managing case*
- *In proper location where it is supposed to be*

I hope this helps when you need it.

Quick Notes for CCU/ICU Nurse Rounds

Purpose: Guide to help you give pertinent and specific information about patient(s) to oncoming nurse(s) caring for admitted patient(s). Rounds per pet should take no more than three to five minutes unless it's a _very_ complicated case.

1. Cage/run number and location (ICU, main Tx area, isolation, IMC, O_2, I-131, runs, etc.)
2. Signalment: name, age, gender, weight, and breed
3. Date and time admitted
4. Chief complaint and/or symptoms (how long)
5. Diagnosis / surgery description and date / procedure description and date / etc.
6. Pertinent medical history, including medications. Vaccine status.
7. Laboratory: pertinent items / diagnostics performed or to be performed
8. Medication(s): pertinent items (general description)
9. Precautions (e.g., wear gloves, neutropenic or chemotherapy, save stool, nonambulatory, etc.)
10. Overview of status: appetite, bowel movement, urination, vomiting (?), mentation, respiration, cardiac concerns, oxygen, etc.
11. Plan: staying, to be discharged (when), if any upcoming procedure or surgery is to be performed
12. Key nursing item(s) (e.g., need pillow, does best on the right side, noise sensitive, etc.)
13. When to alert or call DVM: preset DVM parameters or identifiable change in condition or lab work
14. Note if a caution: describe type of caution (temp, will bite, restraint, all procedures, painful, etc.)
15. Code status: CPR vs. DNR
16. Any changes in treatment plan during the shift (e.g., urinary catheter placed, d/c fluids, change IV vs. oral meds, oxygen start/stop, etc.)

17. Any updates with nursing observations: IV catheter replaced or pulled, temperature high or low, fluid adjustments, neurologic status better/worse, etc.
18. If the family is planning to visit, what time?
19. Identify who in the family is the point person for medical and financial updates.
20. Financial status update: Are charges current and complete? Do we need to collect more funds?
21. TIP: Answer any questions. Be factual. Leave emotion out. Stay focused and pay attention during rounds.

Sample Rounds Format

Patient: _____ Weight: _____lb _____kg
Client: _____ Age: ___ Gender: ___ Breed: ___
Chief Complaint: _____
History: _____
_____
Vaccine Status (current yes or no): _____
Medications or Allergies: _____
_____
Diagnosis: _____
Plan: _____
_____
_____
_____
_____
_____
_____
_____
_____
_____
_____
_____
_____
_____

Code Status: CPR vs. DNR   Financial Status: _____

Feline and Canine Bone Basic Anatomy

Cat Skeletal System

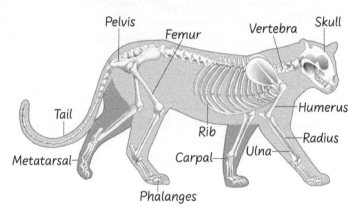

Photo courtesy: Pinterest

ANATOMY OF A DOG

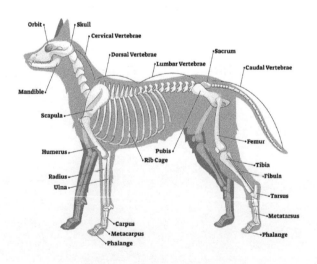

Photo courtesy: Getty Images

Feline and Canine Dental Chart

Adult Feline Dental Anatomy

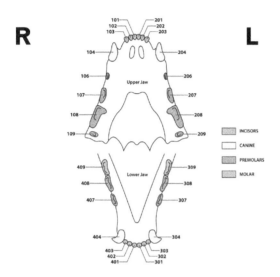

Adult Canine Dental Anatomy

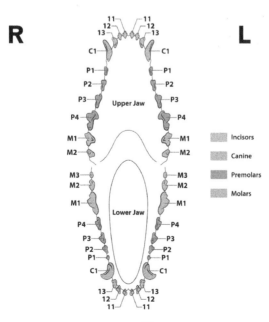

13

Triage: Rapid Trauma Assessment

NOTE: Please use your judgment for the safety and health of you, your patient(s), the client, and the hospital staff before examining the patient. All items listed are not in any particular order and may need to be combined with the medical assessment. You may need to use an assistant or technician to aid you in gathering the following information simultaneously.

All the following items may not be necessary or may need to wait for evaluation by the veterinarian and are in no way limited to the following:

DCAPBTLS

D—Deformities/Distention/ Discoloration

C—Contusions

A—Abrasions

P—Punctures/Penetrations

B—Bleeding/Bruising/Bumps/Burns

T—Tenderness

L—Lacerations

S—Swelling

CMSTP

C—Circulation

M—Motor Function

S—Sensation

T—Temperature

P—Pulse

Vitals = May not include all the following due to the patient's status:
> Weight, TPR, MM, CRT, BP, and SpO$_2$

Head = Head, face, eyes, ears, nose, and mouth
> Check for DCAPBTLS, PLR, symmetry, mucous membrane color, crepitation, drainage, loose or broken teeth, parasites, objects that could cause obstruction, laceration of the tongue, unusual breath odor, and discoloration.

Neck
➤ Check for DCAPBTLS, jugular vein distention, parasites, and crepitation.

Chest
➤ Check for DCAPBTLS, paradoxical motion, parasites, and crepitation. Listen to heart and for breath sounds.

Abdomen
➤ Check for DCAPBTLS, firmness, softness, distention, and parasites.

Pelvis
➤ Check for DCAPBTLS and CMSTP (including tail). Check vulva, penis, and prepuce and scrotum for parasites, symmetry, and/or texture as well as anal sacs.

Extremities
➤ Check for DCAPBTLS and CMSTP. Note feel for pulses while simultaneously listening to the heart.

Spine
➤ Check for DCAPBTLS. Assess tail movement and anal tone.

Triage: Rapid Medical Patient Assessment

NOTE: Please use your judgment for the safety and health of you, your patient(s), the client, and the hospital staff before examining the patient. All items listed are not in any particular order and may need to be combined with the trauma assessment. You may need to use an assistant or technician to aid you in gathering the following information simultaneously.

All the following items <u>may not</u> be necessary or may need to wait for evaluation by the veterinarian and are in <u>no way</u> limited to the following:

- Gather the history of the <u>present</u> illness = **OPQRST**
  - o O—Onset: When did the problem(s) start?
  - o P—Provokes: What aggravated the problem?
  - o Q—Quality: Describe the problem.
  - o R—Radiation: Is the condition associated with anything else?
  - o S—Severity: What is the scale of the condition(s)/problem(s)?
  - o T—Time: How long do you think it's been going on?

- Gather a **SAMPLE** history from the responsible party
  - o S—Signs and symptoms
  - o A—Allergies to medications
  - o M—Medications currently being taken
  - o P—Pertinent present and past history
  - o L—Last oral intake of food or medication
  - o E—Events leading to the current condition

- Conduct a focused physical exam on the area(s) regarding the <u>chief complaint</u>

- Obtain baseline vital signs: may not include all the following:
  - o Weight, TPR, MM, and CRT
  - o Optional (depending on the patient's presentation): BP, ECG, and SpO_2

Dehydration Assessment

*Not all animals will exhibit all signs.

Dehydration	Physical Exam Findings
Euhydrated	Euhydrated (normal)
Mild (~5%)	Minimal loss of skin turgor, semidry mucous membranes, normal eye
Moderate (~8%)	Moderate loss of skin turgor, dry mucous membranes, weak rapid pulses, enophthalmos
Severe (> 10%)	Considerable loss of skin turgor, severe enophthalmos, tachycardia, extremely dry mucous membranes, weak/thready pulses, hypotension, altered level of consciousness

Calculating mcg/kg/min

Equation: wt (kg) × dose (mcg/kg/min) = mcg/min

Breakdown

$$\frac{mcg}{min} \times \frac{ml}{mcg} = \frac{ml}{min} \times \frac{60\ min}{hr} = \frac{ml}{hr}$$

Example: 45 kg patient

Dose: 6 mcg/kg/min

Drug concentration: 1,000 mcg/ml

45 kg × 6 mcg/kg/min = 270 mcg/min

You need to calculate to get the rate as ml/hr.

$$\frac{270\ mcg}{min} \times \frac{ml}{1,000\ mcg} = \frac{0.27\ ml}{min} \times \frac{60\ min}{hr} = \frac{16.2\ ml}{hr}$$

Answer: Set pump to 16 ml/hr

Calculating mcg/kg/hr

Equation: wt (kg) × dose (mcg/kg/min) × concentration (mcg/ml) × time (hr)

Breakdown

$$\frac{kg}{1} \times \frac{mcg}{kg} \times \frac{ml}{mcg} \times \frac{1}{hr} = \frac{ml}{hr}$$

Example: 36 kg patient

Dose: 3 mcg/kg/hr

Drug concentration: 50 mcg/ml

36 kg × 3 mcg/kg/hr = 108 mcg/hr

You need to calculate to get the rate as ml/hr.

$$\frac{36\ kg}{1} \times \frac{3\ mcg}{kg} \times \frac{ml}{50\ mcg} \times \frac{1}{hr} = \frac{2.16\ ml}{hr}$$

Answer: Set pump to 2.16 ml/hr

Calculating mg/kg/day (24 hrs)

You will need to know: wt (kg) - dose (mg/kg/24 hrs) - fluid rate (ml/hr) - volume of fluids in bag

Breakdown

Step 1: <u>ml in bag</u> / rate <u>ml</u> = <u>total hours</u>
hr

Step 2: Total hours × calculated dose (mg/kg/24 hrs) = mg dose

Step 3: Total mg dose / mg/ml concentration of drug = ml to add to bag

Example: 29 kg patient

Dose: 2 mg/kg/day = 58 mg/day

Drug concentration: 5 mg/ml

Hourly fluid rate: 150 ml/hr

Volume of fluids in bag: 1,000 ml (full bag)

You need to calculate to get the rate as ml to add to fluid bag.

Step 1: <u>1,000 ml bag</u> ÷ 150 <u>ml</u> = 6.6 <u>total hours</u>
hr

Step 2: 6.6 total hours × calculated dose (58 mg/day) ÷ 24 hrs = total mg dose = 15.95 mg

Step 3: 15.95 total mg dose ÷ 5 mg/ml concentration of drug = 3.19 ml of drug to add to bag

Answer: Add 3.19 ml of drug to bag. Then set pump to 150 ml/hr, which is the prescribed fluid rate in the above example.

Thoracocentesis (Chest Tap) Supply List

Note: Items are in no particular order. The **DVM** may need options, so be prepared to add or adjust items in this list to their preference and patient needs.

Tip: Have **DVM** plus two support team members. **DVM** will perform the procedure, one team member will restrain the patient, and the second team member will be managing the centesis setup to evacuate the fluid with the **DVM**'s direction.

- ➢ Exam table—preferably in a quiet area to avoid overstimulating patient during procedure
- ➢ (2) 19 g × 3 ¼" butterfly catheter
- ➢ (2) 18 g × 1 ¼" needles and (2) 20 g × 1" needles
- ➢ (2) 18 g (long) catheters
- ➢ (1) three-way stopcock
- ➢ (2) extension sets
- ➢ (1) **LTT** (lavender top tube)
- ➢ (1) **RTT** (red top tube)
- ➢ (1) **WTT** (white top tube)
- ➢ (1) culture swab
- ➢ Lab form(s) to submit sample if applicable
- ➢ (1) 20 cc syringe—Luer lock preferred
- ➢ (1) 60 cc syringe—Luer lock preferred
- ➢ (1) Suction container or bowl to collect and measure fluid in
- ➢ Scrub
- ➢ Alcohol
- ➢ Clippers
- ➢ Ultrasound machine—if available at your practice
- ➢ Wetproof tape to secure extension line to container/bowl
- ➢ Anesthesia monitoring sheet—paper or electronic
- ➢ Multiparameter monitoring equipment (unit with SpO_2, BP, temp, $ETCO_2$, and EKG)

o   Confirm the potential need of the following items with the DVM:

➤ Sterile gloves—confirm size and type (latex vs. nonlatex) for DVM
➤ Sterile gauze
➤ IV catheter in patient
➤ Oxygen source (anesthetic machine)
➤ IV fluids and setup (DVM to prescribe dose and fluid type if applicable)
➤ Sedation or pain medication (if safe and/or required)

Wound Repair / Laceration Supplies

Note: Items are in no particular order. The DVM may need options, so be prepared to add or adjust items in this list to their preference and patient needs:

- ➤ Procedure room and/or table for patient
- ➤ Dilute chlorhexidine solution to cleanse/flush wounds
- ➤ (1) 12 cc curved-tip syringes
- ➤ (3 sizes) Penrose drain
- ➤ (1) Laceration pack—ER surgery minor pack
- ➤ (1) 1 L bag NaCl (saline) used for wound flush
- ➤ (1) 1 L bottle NaCl (saline) used for wound flush
- ➤ (2) 18-gauge needle to puncture saline bottle top for wound rinse
- ➤ (1) three-way stopcock (used for wound flush line)
- ➤ (1) Macro drip set (used for wound flush line)
- ➤ IV Pole—to hang wound flush fluids
- ➤ (1) 18 g cannula tip used for wound flush
- ➤ (1) 2-0 Ethilon suture
- ➤ (1) 3-0 Ethilon suture
- ➤ (1) 10 scalpel blade
- ➤ (1) 15 scalpel blade
- ➤ (1) Skin stapler
- ➤ Chlorhexidine scrub diluted
- ➤ Chlorhexidine solution diluted
- ➤ 3 × 3 sterile gauze
- ➤ Sterile lube—to protect wound while clipping fur
- ➤ Clippers
- ➤ Fenestrated drape—adequate size for wound (if needed)
- ➤ Sterile gloves—confirm size and type (latex vs. nonlatex) for DVM
- ➤ Towels—to absorb saline on floor during procedure

  - o Confirm the potential need of the following items with the DVM:

- IV catheter in patient
- Bandage materials—vet wrap, stretch gauze, cotton roll, Telfa pad, porous tape, etc.
- IV fluids and setup with pump (DVM to prescribe dose and fluid type)
- Sedation and/or anesthesia (if required)—see anesthesia supplies list
- Local anesthetic (if requested)
- Lidocaine jelly for direct wound use
- Oxygen source (anesthetic machine)
- Anesthesia monitoring sheet—paper or electronic
- If anesthetized—multiparameter monitoring equipment (unit with SpO_2, BP, temp, $ETCO_2$, and EKG)
- Clean and prepare cage for patient to recover in
- Enter charges into invoice
- Prepare flow sheet for treatments after procedure

Blocked Cat Supply List

Note: Items are in no particular order. The **DVM** may need options, so be prepared to add or adjust items in this list to their preference and patient needs:

- ➢ Procedure room and/or table for patient
- ➢ (1) 3.5 fr red rubber catheter
- ➢ (1) 5 fr red rubber catheter
- ➢ (1) Slippery Sam catheter
- ➢ (1) Tom Cat catheter (open-ended)
- ➢ (2) Sterile lube pouches
- ➢ (1) Macro drip set
- ➢ (1) Closed urine collection bag
- ➢ (1) **WTT** (white top tube)
- ➢ Lab form to submit sample if applicable
- ➢ (1) 6 cc syringe—to collect samples to run tests
- ➢ (1) 35 cc syringe
- ➢ (1) 3-0 nylon suture
- ➢ (1) 2" vet wrap
- ➢ (1) 1" porous tape
- ➢ (1) Little Herbert—Luer lock adapter
- ➢ Dilute chlorhexidine scrub
- ➢ Clippers
- ➢ Ultrasound machine
- ➢ (2) sterile saline bag (250 ml)—one for flushing bladder during procedure and one for hospitalized u-cath care
- ➢ (3) 60 cc syringes with sterile saline in them
- ➢ (1) Needle holders with scissors
- ➢ (1) Thumb forceps
- ➢ Sterile gloves—confirm size and type (latex vs. nonlatex) for **DVM**

  - o Confirm the potential need of the following items with the **DVM**:

- ➤ IV catheter in patient
- ➤ Tape (wetproof or porous) to secure u-cath line to pet's tail
- ➤ IV fluids and setup with pump (DVM to prescribe dose and fluid type)
- ➤ Sedation (if required)
- ➤ Oxygen source (anesthetic machine)
- ➤ Anesthesia monitoring sheet—paper or electronic
- ➤ If anesthetized—multiparameter monitoring equipment (unit with SpO_2, BP, temp, $ETCO_2$, and EKG)
- ➤ Clean and prepare cage for patient to recover in
- ➤ Enter charges into invoice
- ➤ Prepare flow sheet for treatments after procedure
- ➤ Radiology setup for post-placement images

Basic Anesthesia Supply List

Note: Items are in no particular order. The DVM may need options, so be prepared to add or adjust items in this list to their preference and patient needs:

- Procedure room and/or table for patient
- Anesthesia machine and/or ventilator setup and pressure checked
- Anesthesia scavenger system setup and confirmed functional
- Anesthesia monitoring sheet—paper or electronic
- Endotracheal (ET) tubes—three sizes that may fit your patient. Do cuff leak test to ensure patency and safety.
- Laryngoscope, with properly sized blade attachment, to help with placement of ET tube
- Sterile lube packet to help with placement of ET tube
- Empty clean syringe for air to inflate cuff on ET tube (3 cc–20 cc, depending on cuff size)
- Tie to secure ET tube
- 3 × 3 dry gauze—to hold tongue during intubation
- Premed agents: DVM to prescribe drug(s) and dosage. Document on anesthesia form.
- Anesthetic agents: DVM to prescribe drug(s) and dosage. Document on anesthesia form.
- 2 towels or bedding for table to place under and over patient
- Warm water blanket to place under patient for thermal regulation—if available
- IV fluid warmer—if available
- Bair Hugger or other warm air unit to place over your patient for thermal regulation—if available
- IV catheter placed in patient
- IV fluid setup with pump—if appropriate for your patient. Confirm with DVM.

- ➢ Multiparameter monitoring equipment (unit with SpO_2, BP, temp, $ETCO_2$, and EKG)
- ➢ Artificial tear ointment or other eye lubricant to keep eyes moistened during procedure
- ➢ Gas anesthetic agent (isoflurane or sevoflurane)—make sure the anesthesia vaporizer is full
- ➢ Emergency drugs—have precalculated and readily available during procedure

Anesthetic Risk Classification

According to the American Society of Anesthesiologists

ASA 1
Minimal risk
Normal, healthy animal; no underlying disease

ASA 2
Slight risk, minor disease present
Animal with slight to mild systemic disturbance, animal able to compensate
Neonate or geriatric animals, obese

ASA 3
Moderate risk, obvious disease present
Animal with moderate systemic disease or disturbances, mild clinical signs
Anemia, moderate dehydration, fever, low-grade heart murmur, or cardiac disease

ASA 4
High risk, significantly compromised by disease
Animals with preexisting systemic disease or disturbances of a severe nature
Severe dehydration, shock, uremia, toxemia, high fever, uncompensated heart disease, uncompensated diabetes, pulmonary disease, emaciation

ASA 5
Extreme risk, moribund
Surgery often performed in desperation on animal with life-threatening systemic disease
Advanced cases of heart, kidney, liver, or endocrine disease; profound shock; severe trauma; pulmonary embolism; terminal malignancy

The Five Rights of Medication

1. Right patient to be treated
2. Right drug to be provided
3. Right dose prescribed
4. Right time to be given
5. Right route to be administered
6. (Bonus) Right documentation in medical record

General Patient Assessment

SAMPLE History

S—Signs and symptoms: What is the presenting complaint?

A—Allergies: Any known drug, food, or environmental allergies

M—Medications: List all medications (prescribed, over-the-counter, supplement, etc.)

P— Past medical history: Any pertinent and historic medical information

L— Last oral intake: Food and medication (dose and time of last meal and meds)

E— Events leading up to: What was patient doing just before the issue started?

Basic Descriptions for Patient Assessment

Attitude

- BAR (bright, alert, responsive)
- QAR (quiet, alert, responsive)
- Sleeping
- Painful
- Depressed
- Sedate
- Obtunded
- Comatose

Condition

- Stable
- No change
- Improved
- Deteriorating

Respiratory Character

- Relaxed
- Panting
- Labored
- Deep
- Shallow
- Dyspneic

Neuro Signs
- Tremors
- Twitching
- Seizure
- Ataxic
- Anisocoria
- Nystagmus

Mucous Membranes
- Pink
- Light pink
- Pale
- Injected
- Muddy
- Icteric
- Gray
- Cyanotic
- White

Quantity
0 = Nothing produced, +1 = 25% produced, +2 = 50% produced, +3 = 75% produced, +4 = 100% or more produced

Nerve Agent Exposure Patient Assessment

SLUDGE

S—Salivation and/or seizure
L—Lacrimation: Tearing/watery eyes
U—Urination: Incontinence vs. straining
D—Defecation: Loose stool vs. constipation
G—Gastrointestinal pain and/or gas
E—Emesis: Vomiting and/or dry heaving

Painful Patient Assessment

OPQRST

O—Onset: When were symptoms first noted?

P—Provokes: What makes it worse?

Q—Quality: Describe the symptoms.

R—Radiates: Any symptoms associated

S—Severity: Rate the pain on a scale of 0–10.

T— Time: How long, and if worse, is it at a particular time of day or after activity?

Respiratory Patient Assessment

PASTE

P—Provokes: What makes it worse?

A—Associated pain: Any additional symptoms

S—Sputum: Coughing up any phlegm. What color?

T— Tired: Does patient get tired easily (e.g., takes a few steps then needs to rest)?

E— Exercise intolerance: Patient no longer able to perform normal play and activity.

Charge Capture Tips

Hospitalized Patients

Tip: Have a routine as to how you approach charges to ensure charges aren't missed or duplicated.

Confirm date and DVM managing the case for the shift and/or day.

Proceed to ensure all items have been properly entered into invoice and that they match the treatment flow sheet.

- Hospitalization
- IV catheter(s) and fluid setup
- Fluids
- Additives
- CRIs
- Infusion pumps
- Injections: pain
- Injections: antibiotics
- Injections: gastrointestinal
- Injections: chemotherapy agents
- Oral medications
- Topical medications
- Eye medications
- Ear medications
- Lab tests: in-house
- Lab tests: outside labs
- Diagnostic imaging: radiology, ultrasound, CT scan, MRI, etc.
- Wound care and/or bandage
- Catheter care
- Oxygen
- Physical therapy
- Recumbency care

- Heat support
- Tube feeding
- Procedure: centesis, central line, etc.
- If pet's quality of life deteriorates, consider following charges:
  - Euthanasia
  - Care of remains
  - Special memorial items: paw print and the like

Patient Discharge Tips

Confirm the following tasks have been completed:

- Finalize invoice and ensure all charged are accurate and complete
- All personal belongings are gathered
  - Collar, leash, harness, carrier, bedding, toys, food, meds, etc.
- Home care instructions are correct and complete
  - Name and gender are correct on all comments
  - Drug info and frequency are correct (Q12H vs. Q8H)
  - DVM and medical team info is correct
  - Note when next dose of medications is due
  - Inform client when pet last ate
  - Inform client when pet had last BM or urination
  - Inform client if pet is nauseous
  - Inform client if pet is still feeling drowsy and how to be safe
- Medications are made, stored, and labeled with precautions
  - Refrigerate, give with food, cause drowsiness, shake well, etc.
  - Proper-sized syringe is provided for liquid medications
- Remove IV catheter(s) and/or central lines
- Remove monitoring device attachments
  - BP cuff, ECG electrodes, continuous temp probe, etc.
- Pet is clean and free of debris
  - Surgical incision is not bloody
  - Genitals have no urine or feces
  - Face is clear of nasal, ear, or eye discharge
- Place a clean e-collar if appropriate
- Sling or harness if appropriate
- Confirm next, or all necessary, follow-up visits are prescheduled
  - Drain removal
  - Bandage or splint change or removal

- o Suture or staple removal vs. incision check
- o Radiographs
- o Follow-up lab tests

Secondary Items After Pet Is Discharged

- Clean and disinfect cage and reset for next patient
- Remove pet from white board (posted, printed, or electronic)
- Recycle care card
- Clean dishes used
- Place dirty laundry to be cleaned
- Replace miscellaneous items
  - o Fluid and syringe pumps
  - o Monitoring equipment
  - o Medical supplies: oxygen, nebulization, glucose meters, etc.

Temperature Conversions

Celsius to Fahrenheit: (Celsius) × (9/5) + 32 = temp
Example: 38 Celsius × 9/5 = 68.4 + 32 = 100.4 F

Fahrenheit to Celsius: Fahrenheit - 32 × 5/9 = temp
Example: 101.8 - 32 = 69.5 × 5/9 = 38.6 C

Weight Conversions

1lb = 453.6 g
1lb = 0.453 kg
1lb = 16 oz
1 oz = 28.35 g
1 kg = 2.2 lb
1 g = 1,000 mg
1 mg = 1,000 ug (mcg)
1 mg = 0.001 g
1 ug = 0.001 mg
1 ug = 0.000001 g

lb = pound
kg = kilogram
g = gram
ug (mcg) = microgram
oz = ounce

Volume Conversions

1 drop (gt) = 0.06 ml
15 drops (gtt) = 1 ml (cc)
1 teaspoon (tsp) = 5 ml
1 tablespoon (tbs) = 15 ml
2 tbs = 30 ml
1 ounce (oz) = 30 ml
1 teacup = 180 ml
6 oz = 180 ml
1 cup = 240 ml
8 oz = 1 cup

Unit Conversions

Factor Given	Unit Wanted	To convert to unit wanted, multiply factor by
lb	kg	0.45
kg	lb	2.2
kg	g	1,000
g	mg	1,000
oz	g	28.35
oz	lb	16
g	ug	1,000,000
kg	mg	1,000,000
mg/kg	mg/lb	0.4536
mg/g	mg/lb	453.6
kcal/kg	kcal/lb	0.4536
kcal/lb	kcal/kg	2.2046
mg/kg	%	0.001
mg/g	%	0.1

Basic Drug Routes and Frequencies

Routes:
PO (per os) = by mouth
NPO (nil per os) = nothing by mouth
PC (post cibum) = after food
PT = per tube (e.g., feeding tube)
OU (oculus uterque) = both eyes
OD (oculus dexter) = right eye
OS (oculus sinister) = left eye
AU (aures unitas) = both ears
AD (auris dextra) = right ear
AS (auris sinistra) = left ear
IV = intravenously
IM = intramuscularly
SQ = subcutaneously

Frequencies:
SID (semel in die) = once daily (Q24H)
BID (bis in die) = twice daily (Q12H)
TID (ter in die) = three times daily (Q8H)
QID (quater in die) = four times daily (Q6H)
PRN (pro re nata) = as needed
EOD = every other day (Q48H)

References

Battaglia, Andrea M. 2001. *Small Animal Emergency and Critical Care: A Manual for the Veterinary Technician.*

Edwards, N. Joel. 1993. *ECG Manual for the Veterinary Technician.*

Hendrix and Sirois. 2007. *Laboratory Procedures for Veterinary Technicians.* 5th ed.

Jack, Watson, and Donovan. 2008. *Veterinary Technician Daily Reference Guide.* 2nd ed.

Kirk, Bistner, and Ford. 1964. *Handbook of Veterinary Procedures and Emergency Treatment.* 6th ed.

Lake, Terry. 2004. *Dosage Calculations for Veterinary Nurses and Technicians.*

Macintire, Drobatz, Haskins, and Saxon. 2005. *Small Animal and Critical Care Medicine.*

McCurnin. 1998. *Clinical Textbook for Veterinary Technicians.* 4th ed.

Merrill, Linda. 2012. *Small Animal Internal Medicine for Veterinary Technicians and Nurses.*

Plunkett, Signe J. 2001. *Emergency Procedures for the Small Animal Veterinarian.* 2nd ed.

Shade, Bruce R. 2007. *EMT—Intermediate Textbook.* 3rd ed.

Swaim and Henderson. 1990. *Small Animal Wound Management.*

Thurmon, Tranquilli, and Benson. 1999. *Essentials of Small Animal Anesthesia and Analgesia.*

Tracy, Diane L. 2000. *Small Animal Surgical Nursing.* 3rd ed.

Wanamaker and Pettes. 2000. *Applied Pharmacology for the Veterinary Technician.* 2nd ed.

Photos of the author at work

Assisting with Endoscopy

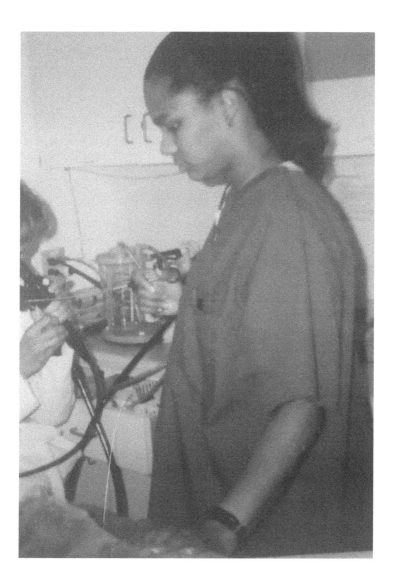

Assisting with Laparoscopic Liver Biopsy

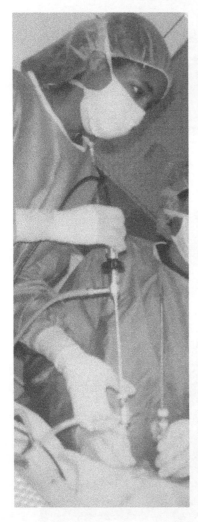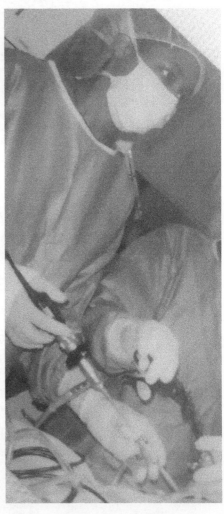

Surgical Assisting

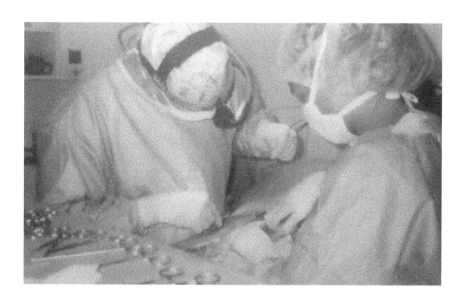

Patient Care at Its Finest

She wouldn't relax unless someone was lying with her.
Of course I had to take one for the team!

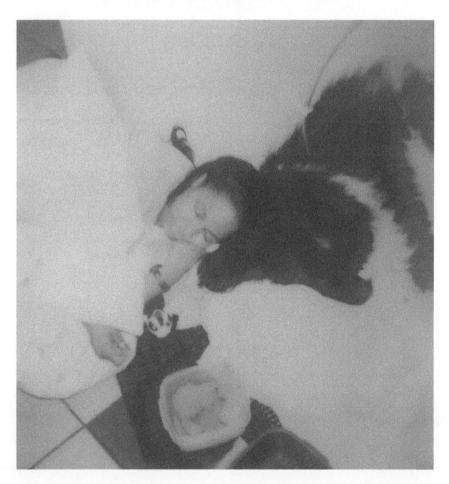

Diagnostic Imaging—Gamma Camera

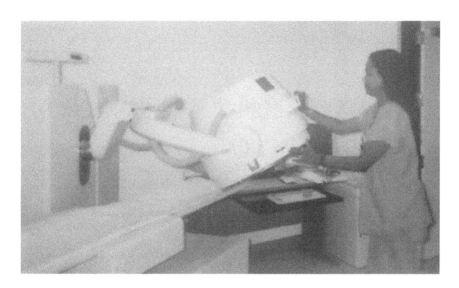

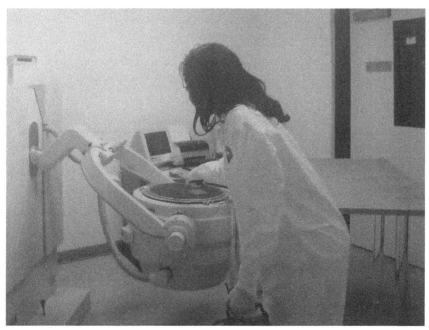

Linear Accelerator—Radiation Therapy

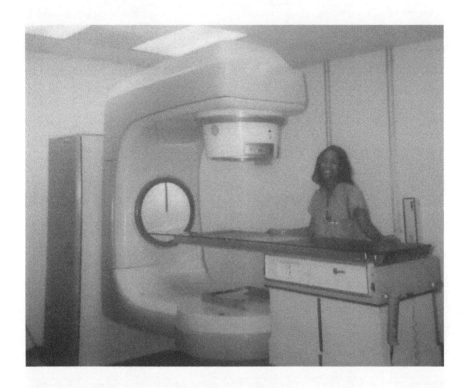

Diagnostic Imaging—CT Scan

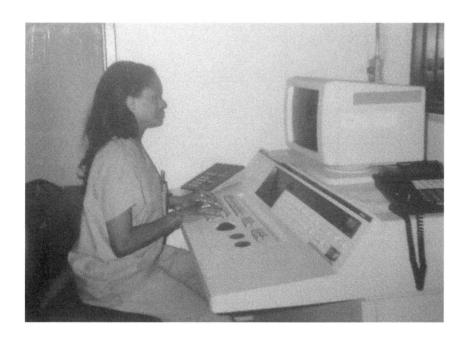

Prepping for Surgery

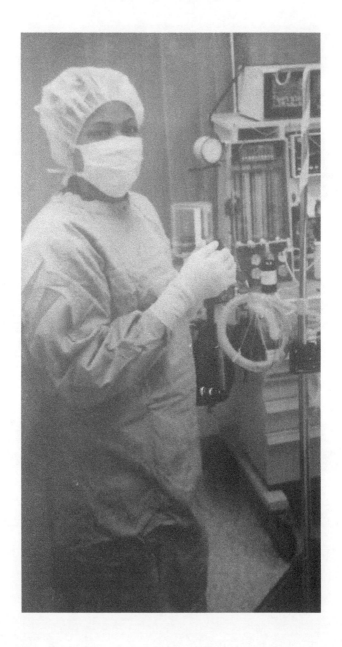

Orthopedic Surgical Assisting

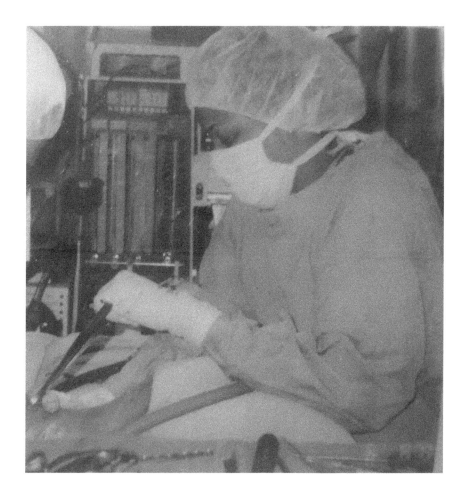

Bandaging Front Limb

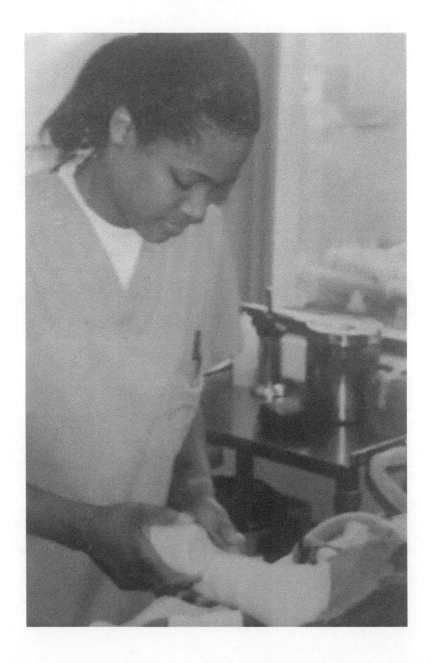

Suturing Post-Op Orthopedic Case

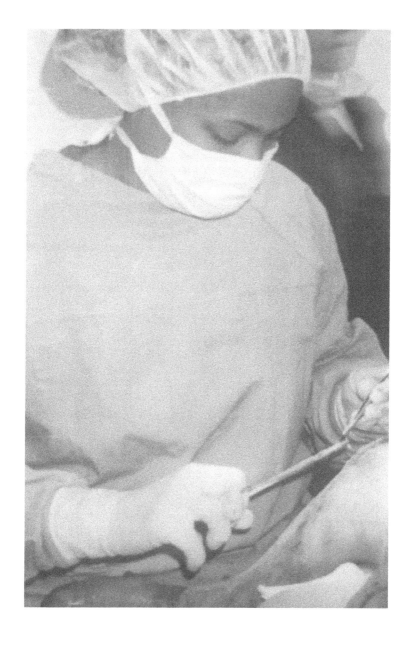

Doppler Blood Pressure

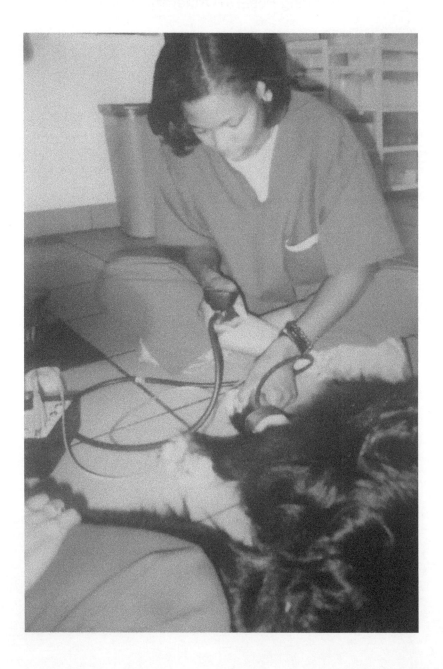

Guinea Pig Bandage Change

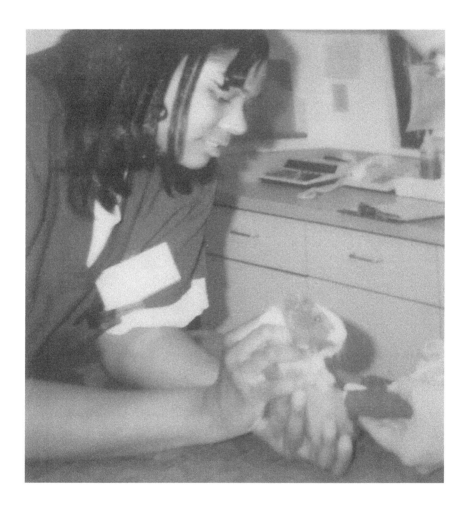

Documenting Treatment on the Medical Record

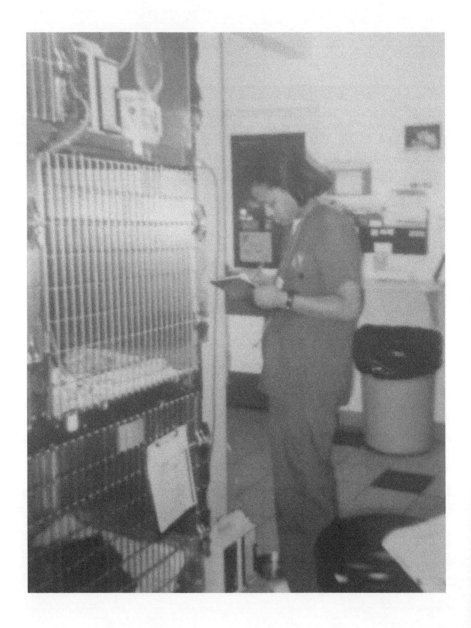

Jugular Catheter Placement
Central Line

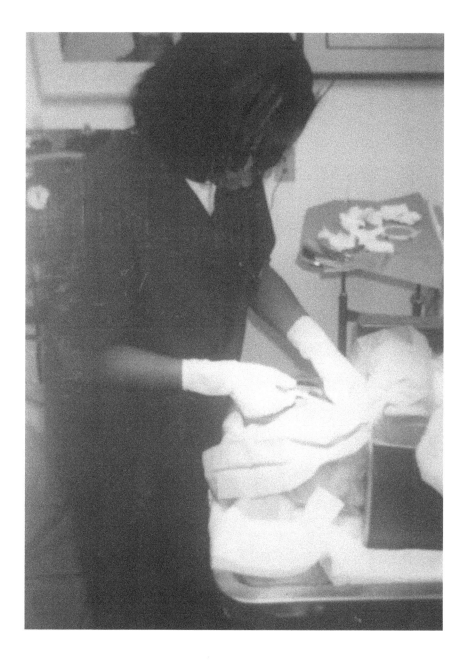

Index

Lightning Source UK Ltd.
Milton Keynes UK
UKHW012050120821
388784UK00008B/452/J

9 781664 187474